Cordyceps Sinensis

Immune and Stamina Booster

KATE GILBERT UDALL

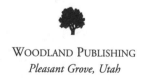

WOODLAND PUBLISHING
Pleasant Grove, Utah

ISBN 1-58054-047-3

Table of Contents

Cordyceps Sinensis: An Introduction

In the 1990s, mainstream medicine has seen a change in its willingness to accept the legitimacy of natural therapies. In fact, much recent scientific confirmation has been established for the effectiveness of natural therapies in curing disease and maintaining health. This phenomenon has been manifest in the use of botanical agents for treatments ranging from annoying skin problems to life-threatening diseases such as cancer, heart conditions and AIDS. Many practitioners are repeatedly turning to alternative forms of treatments and combinations of alternative and traditional medicine.

Recent medical inquiry into alternative health therapies has supported the notion that healthful living along with appropriate supplements is an effective way to avoid and treat many ailments and illnesses. Subsequently, the market for herbal supplements has boomed, and the Western world is beginning to enjoy the benefits of herbs that have been long used in China.

Making use of the benefits of health through the consumption of herbs is important, as most of us would probably agree that the key to well-being is good health. Feeling strong and energetic is a result of good health that makes life more enjoyable for everyone. Our energy and endurance levels, and thus, our health and quality of life, can be directly influenced by our immune system. A balanced and healthy immune system is central to the body's ability to defend against infections; anything we can do to strengthen our immune system will help to assure our well-being and longevity. Dr. Richard Bennett has said,

"It's in our ability to create a really healthy immune system that I think represents the greatest potential in gains in human health in the world. If we can do something to make us all just a little bit more healthier, there's going to be less disease and less suffering.

As research has shown, one of the things we can do to stop the natural decline of the immune system is to add supplements to our daily health regimens. *Cordyceps sinensis* is an ancient tonic herb now available in supplement form which has been shown to aid immune function, among other things. In Chinese medicine, *Cordyceps sinensis* is used to reinforce what is called the body's vital energy source. This means it will give you increased levels of stamina and endurance along with enhancing your immune system's ability to fight disease. It also helps nourish the lungs and kidneys and replenish sperm. Biological activity that has been associated with *Cordyceps sinensis* includes the following:

- Strengthening immune function
- Anti-tumor activity
- Enhancing stamina and endurance
- Anti-viral activity
- Increasing longevity
- Resisting respiratory infection (colds/flu, etc.)
- Controlling liver and kidney disfunction
- Improving heart function

This booklet will help you understand how *Cordyceps sinensis* and some complementary herbs can help increase the efficacy of your immune system, improve your levels of stamina and endurance, as well as how you can benefit from other functions of these herbs. Recent research will be presented and discussed supporting what has been known in Chinese medicine all along—that *Cordyceps sinensis* really can make a difference in how you feel and perform.

Cordyceps Sinensis and the Immune System

Many of us have partially suppressed immune systems resulting from poor nutrition, inadequate mineral intake and/or environmental toxins. Often with the natural process of aging, proper immune function can falter even more. Important biological levels of free radical scavenging enzymes are reduced as we pass age 40. This loss has a major impact on our free radical defense mechanisms making us more prone to degenerative diseases. Diet and exercise will always play an important role in our good health and fitness plan, but problems associated with the loss of gene function occur when we age. *Cordyceps sinensis*, when taken in the right manner can help reduce this loss and its associated problems.

Cordyceps Sinensis in Traditional Chinese Medicine

Knowing about the origins of *Cordyceps sinensis* and the role it plays in Chinese medicine helps us understand how the herb works. According to traditional Chinese medicine, disease is thought to develop as a result of a decline in the Zhang (the general resistance of the body.) When this occurs, the causative agents of a disease—what we now call invading pathogenic factors—are able to take hold in the body and bring about an illness. The decline in the general resistance of the body results in failure in homeostasis, which is the normal balance of the body. Many health problems, including poor immune function, are a result of this imbalance.

The herbs which replenished the Zhang were first known as the upper class herbs and were reserved for the rich and the aristocracy. They were used to support weakening health and during certain periods of Chinese history, you were put to death if you were caught cultivating the precious herbs without the permission of the Emperor. *Cordyceps sinensis*, as an ancient tonic herb, is one of the upper class herbs. Around 2700 B.C., these herbs were classified as multi-functional and recommended as body-supporting agents. Tonics, such as *Cordyceps sinensis*, are thought to strengthen the body and restore various functions or homeostasis leading to a balance in the body.

Cordyceps sinensis is one of the most valued medicinal fungi (Shimitsu 1978) in all of Chinese medicine and among the most potent. In Chinese it is called "Winter warm summer grass." It is naturally found in the highlands of China, Tibet and Nepal. In early spring when the snow is just melting, people crawl on the ground to search for the smaller that finger size mushroom.

In this modern scientific time, Cordyceps can be cultivated for higher and purer harvest. It has traditionally been used in China to include the relief of bronchial inflammation; treatment of chronic bronchitis, insomnia, hypertension, pneumonia, emphysema and tuberculosis; relief of exhaustion; debilitation following illness; anemia; night sweats; and cough. Benefits recorded in Chinese medicine have also included: improvement of lung and kidney function; phlegm reduction, cough suppressant; and blood coagulation. Modern medicine has reported these uses: effects on body temperature, immunity, sedation, and anticonvulsion. *Cordyceps sinensis* is known to decrease hypertension, and oxygen consumption in the cardiac muscles and improve the blood vessel system. It has been helpful in curing asthma and other respiratory ailments.

Cordyceps has properties similar to ginseng; both are used to strengthen the body after exhaustion.

Cordyceps sinensis is also typically used to reinforce what is called the *qii*—or the body's vital energy. Sluggish vital energy levels can be a result of an imbalance in the body characterized by frequent colds, infections, fluid retention, coldness, pallor, or a slow pulse. Other associated symptoms may include, feverishness, night sweats, thirst, dry mouth, or a fast pulse.

Biological Activity of Cordyceps Sinensis

Important properties of *Cordyceps sinensis* include action on the immune system, anti-asthmatic effect, action on male sex hormones, and the ability to act as a smooth muscle relaxant. And numerous reports have shown an effect on the growth of cancer cells in vitro (in the laboratory). It helps nourish the lungs and kidneys and replenish sperm. Studies have demonstrated the amazing multi-functional action of this important traditional medicine.

These biological actions of *Cordyceps sinensis* are due to a number of substances in its makeup. One of these constituents, called Cordycepin (cordycepin-3'-deoxyadenosine), is found in very high concentrations in the fungus. There are a number of other important substances present, including Galactomannan polysaccharides, fatty and amino acids, b1-3 glucans and some pyranosides. Although many of the reports have been animal or in vitro studies there are still a great number of human clinical and epidemiological studies to support its biological activity.

Of the other components that are found in *Cordyceps sinensis* the polysaccharides are probably the next most important of the active substances. Cordyceps has been shown to have a number of polysaccharides in their structure. Polysaccharides are substances like cellulose -made up of a lot sugars joined together but indigestible, ie, a fibre. One of these polysaccharides is b1-3 Glucan, a very powerful biological response modifier. These modifiers are substances that alter the degree to which the immune system responds to a stimulus. The remainder of this section will discuss specific biological actions associated with *Cordyceps sinensis* and present relevant research.

Strengthening Immune Function

Possibly the most important biological feature of *Cordyceps sinensis* is its immunomodulatory effect. Since the 1960's there have been numerous scientific papers written about the wide range of biological activities associated with extracts of Cordyceps hyphae. Between 1991 and 1997, 14 of the 33 more recent studies have been articles related to the immunomodulatory effects of *Cordyceps sinensis*. Cell mediated immune responses and cancer therapy studies have substantiated earlier claims as to Cordyceps being a powerful immune regulator. In vitro studies have demonstrated a significant effect on human T-helper cell function (Zhen, 1992). Cordyceps enhances immunity by increasing the activity of T-cells.

Besides helping the body restore a partially suppressed immune system, which can more effectively ward off illnesses, *Cordyceps sinensis* has been shown to have powerful protective effects in autoimmune diseases. Chen et al, 1993, found that Cordyceps inhibited anti-ds-DNA production, giving it great potential in treating human systemic lupus erythematosus (SLE) —an important autoimmune disease with multiple organ system involvement.

Convincing scientific studies are also available regarding cordycepin, a derivative found in *Cordyceps sinensis*. In 1989, and later in 1991, two independent groups reported on the possibility of reducing the spread of AIDS through the action of cordycepin. Montefiori et al (1989), reported that cordycepin inhibited the action of Human Immunodeficiency Virus Type 1 reverse transcriptase, and hence the spread of HIV infection. Reverse transcriptase is an enzyme that viruses use to decode the message from DNA in the opposite direction to normal. This allows the virus to make a lot more proteins from the same piece of DNA. If you disable this enzyme then the virus is not able to produce the proteins it needs to grow and infect the host cells. Essentially this process would inhibit the spread of HIV infection.

Two years later Muller et al., (1991) reporting in the journal *Biochemistry,* also presented results on the inhibitory effects of cordycepin in respect to its action on HIV Type 1 reverse transcriptase and subsequent viral infection. Although these reports do not provide the miracle answer to the spread of AIDS, they show that progress is being made. It would be necessary to carry out controlled clinical trials, in humans, before the true value of these studies could be determined.

Interestingly, there is another phytochemical, curcumin, from turmeric, that has also been shown to have inhibitory effects on HIV type 1 integrase (Muzumder, 1995), another important HIV enzyme, and in a limited clinical trial curcumin has been shown to have a normalizing effect on CD4/CD8 ratio. This is important in autoimmunity as this ratio is related to immunosuppression, which can contribute to the progression of the disease.

Antitumor Activity

Researchers report that *Cordyceps sinensis* is able to control the division of cancer cells, delay the diffusion of cancer cells and increase the engulfing abilities of T-cells and in the human body, strengthening the fight against cancer. Various bioactive components are contained in fungi of the genus Cordyceps. In 1950, the derivative cordycepin (mentioned above) was first isolated by Cunningham et al. (Cunningham et al., 1950). Although a number of the chemical components of Cordyceps have been shown to have regulatory properties, the derivative cordycepin, which constitutes 32% of the fungus by weight, is the major bioactive substance.

Reported biological activities of cordycepin include:

- Inhibition of DNA and RNA
- Enhancement of cell differentiation
- Restructuring of cytoskeleton in cells
- Inhibition of protein kinase activity
- Anti-tumor activity on bladder, colon and lung carcinoma
- Inhibition of the infection and reverse transcriptase activity of human immunodeficiency virus type 1 (Montefiori et al.; 1989)

And in 1983, a polysaccharide isolated from Cordyceps was shown to prevent the growth of sarcoma in mice. (Ukai et al 1983) Other polysaccharides have also been reported as anti-tumor agents (Ohmari et al, 1986 and Yanada, 1984). It appears that cordycepin and polysaccharides join forces to potentially have impressive cancer fighting capabilities (Kuo, W.Y. et al., 1989).

Kuo, Y.H. et al. (1994), extracted *Cordyceps sinensis* and separated it into a number of different structures. They found that substances other than the polysaccharides or cordycepin were also capable of killing a number of cancer cells in vitro. These b-Glucans are found in a number of yeasts, fungi and some plants. They are found in *Aloe vera* and are what give it its great wound healing properties. The same substance is found in oats and is the substance responsible for the great skin effects that are associated with an oatmeal mask. Most importantly, b-Glucan is the substance that is found in some mushrooms, one being the source of Lentinan, a very important anti-cancer adjuvant therapy in Japan, where it is a registered therapeutic. Its efficacy was determined after a number of clinical trials (Taguchi et al., 1985).

Cancer cytotoxicity studies have determined, then, that there has been and still is a very definite interest in the use of *Cordyceps sinensis* in the future adjuvant therapy of human cancer. One human clinical trial carried out in China had very encouraging results and it is likely that we will continue to see more work in this area in the future. In this clinical trial performed at the First Affiliated Hospital, Guangzhou University of Traditional Chinese Medicine, 36 patients with advanced breast and lung cancer were treated with *Cordyceps sinensis* capsules and had significant improvement in cell mediated immunity with an associated improvement in the quality of life. These results affirm that Cordyceps could be used as an adjuvant in cancer therapy.

Two recent reports by Chen (1997) in *Life Science*, and Tedone (1996) in the journal *European Journal of Cancer* have set the scene for more controlled studies and will undoubtedly generate interest in mainstream Western science. Perhaps in a few years we will see Cordyceps being used in the Western world to the same degree as other herbs are currently used.

Enhancing Stamina and Endurance

Another area of interest in relationship to the use of *Cordyceps sinensis* is that of stamina and endurance. *Cordyceps sinensis* is thought to increase energy by raising the levels of plasma cortisol, thereby increasing the function of plasma cortex and increasing secretion levels of the adrenal gland. This enhances the function of the adrenal gland and strengthens your vital energy. The herb also breaks down lactic acid and acetinic acid—the waste matter in muscles—which makes you less tired during times of stress and exertion and increases motion potential.

Most athletes are very conscious of their diet and how it effects their performance. A careful watch of nutrition is vital to athletes and non-athletes alike. Remember, prolonged intensive exertion can take its toll, overtraining syndrome (OS) and chronic fatigue (CF), being good examples of this. In OS and CF, the suppression of the body's immune system is a major contributor. This is brought about by complex deficits that occur in the body during prolonged or repeated physical stress. Glycogen deficit, catabolic/anabolic imbalances, amino acid imbalance, autonomic imbalance and neuroendocrine imbalance can all result in a counter-regulatory shift in the endocrine system and this contributes to OS and CF. Supplements, such as Cordyceps can work to help the body achieve the balance it needs for healthy function.

Cordyceps recently caught public attention in 1993 when a group of previously mediocre Chinese runners proceeded to break nine world records in World Outdoor Track and Field Championships in Germany. After all the tests for anabolic steroids and the like were completed, and all the tests were found to be negative, the International Federations had only the testimonies of the team and the coach that they had used a Chinese herbal formula. What were they reported to be taking?—a mixture of herbs including Cordyceps.

So how can this tonic herb help you reach peak fitness and increase your stamina? Well, nutritionally Cordyceps will act as a synergist with your other dietary vitamin supplements, reinforcing your immune system and allowing you to recover more quickly during times of stress or after prolonged exertion. This feature of recovery is very important to athletes who will experience a form of immune suppression as a result of physical exertion, "the overtraining syndrome." This immune suppression, while complex in its etiology, results mainly from a counter regulatory shift in the neuroendocrine system. As Cordyceps sinensis is reputed to stimulate the reticuloendothelial and endocrine systems resulting in its stress-reducing effects (Huang, 1993), it is not surprising that Cordyceps extracts can afford protection against overtraining syndrome (OS).

One study, reported by Tang et al. (1986), adds further support to the protective role of Cordyceps in OS, here it was shown that Cordyceps sinensis was able to oppose the immunosuppressive effect of cortisol injections. Cortisol is an adrenal hormone released during catabolic stress that is involved in muscle degradation. If you can reduce the suppressive, catabolic action of cortisol you drive the endocrine system toward anabolism, the building of muscle, which involves protein synthesis and hence nitrogen balance. These two things are very important to performance and recovery after stress.

During an endurance event the muscle and liver glycogen

stores of an athlete become depleted and as much as 15 percent of the energy requirement during that event must be met by muscle degradation. This muscle loss leads to deterioration in muscle recovery and eventually performance. Hence, the elite athlete needs to control catabolism and protect the neuroendocrine system to reduce the occurrence of overtraining syndrome and chronic fatigue—a task, among many, that *Cordyceps sinensis* is ideally suited to.

These effects of *Cordyceps sinensis* make this Chinese herb a factor in achieving higher levels of energy, stamina and endurance desirable for serious athletes and non-athletes alike.

Antiviral and Antibacterial Activity

Cordyceps sinensis has two derivatives—cordycepin, which has already been mentioned, and Corceps acid and cordycepin—which work to resist staphylococcus and other bacillus bacteria strains. Cordyceps has also been shown to resist epidermal and ascites warts.

Cordycepin or 3'-deoxyadenosine is a powerful analogue of adenosine, one of the purine bases that goes into making DNA and RNA. Cordycepin is also a known polyadenylation inhibitor. Polyadenylation is the process used by the cells of the body to move messenger RNA from the nucleus to the cell cytoplasm (Kletzien, 1980). This is necessary for protein synthesis to occur and hence its inhibition will lead to disruption of synthesis. It is this feature that gives cordycepin its powerful anti-viral properties.

Increasing Longevity

Frequently the oxidative stress caused by free radicals results in what we refer to as the "aging process." While aging is inevitable, may of us hasten its outcome by not protecting ourselves, and thus, we age prematurely. The early onset of fatigue, respiratory disorders, diabetes, heart disease, and other problems, can result from free-radical destruction. The damage done by the free radical process results in a compromised immune system that can be minimized by taking herbs such as *Cordyceps sinensis*.

Immune function is often compromised as important biological levels of free radical scavenging enzymes are reduced. Thus, our defense mechanisms make us more prone to illness and degenerative diseases. Besides this hormone production also declines. For example, the circulating levels of Dehydroepiandosterone (DHEA) are known to be lessening from age 25, as does the production of the sex hormones in both males and females. Add to this the numerous environmental hormone disrupters that we are constantly exposed to and it is not surprising to find the large amount of immune disfunction that we see around us. Using *Cordyceps sinensis* as a supplement puts off aging and maintains health by eliminating free radicals in the human body and reducing the damage to biochemical processes of the body.

Resisting Respiratory Problems (Colds/Flu etc.)

The anti-asthmatic property of *Cordyceps sinensis* is one that requires some further comment. A study published by the Taiwan Pediatric Association in April 1996 reported the benefits of *Cordyceps sinensis* in the treatment of asthma and allergic rhinitis. The protective effect of *Cordyceps sinensis* in asthma is in part due to its action as a smooth muscle relaxant. Bronchodilators like Ventolin™ act to relax bronchial smooth muscle and thereby dilate the bronchioles allowing easier breathing. This action, however, only reduces the acute symptoms during an asthma attack.

Preventative treatment in asthma requires the use of anti-inflammatories to reduce the incidence of attack and is the reason why corticosteroids are used. Inhaled corticosteroids give an improved clinical control of asthma by reducing lung inflammation and decreasing airway reactivity. *Cordyceps sinensis*, because of its powerful immunological effects, can also assist in reducing airway reactivity and inflammatory responses, a further reason for its effectiveness in respiratory illness.

Controlling Liver and Kidney Dysfunction

Cordyceps has been shown to protect liver and kidneys and improves lung function. One of the ways it protects the liver is by mediating chronic renal insufficiency, reducing serum creatinine and BUN (Cheng, 1992), and in chronic hepatitis B. In a clinical trial, 33 patients suffering with chronic hepatitis B were given *Cordyceps sinensis* daily. All patients treated were found to have improved liver function and correction of the inversion of albumin to globulin ratio.

Cordyceps also appears to work positively on the liver in times of stress and energy production. Manabe et al (1996), examined the effect of *Cordyceps sinensis* on liver function with special reference to energy production. They found that the supplementation of *Cordyceps sinensis* caused an increase in the energy state of the liver. This was character-ized by the activation of the mitochondrial respiratory transport chain, which leads to a greater energy output and increased ATP levels.

It was also observed that this increased energy produc-tion was not accompanied by a change in intracellular pH. This indicated that normoxic conditions were present in the liver and more importantly they were able to demonstrate that the use of *Cordyceps sinensis* extracts had no toxic side effects. The liver energy enhancing function of *Cordyceps sinensis* is also quite important in the context of perfor-mance, as liver glycogenolysis is a necessity if muscle degra-dation is to be reduced during an endurance event. *Cordyceps sinensis* is also known to potentiate the action of adrenaline, thereby increasing blood glucose levels.

Improving Heart Function

Cordyceps sinensis is known to have the following effects on the heart and cerebral vessels: decreases glycerin trilau-rate, lowers cholesterol and B-lipoprotein levels, prevents thrombosis, resists arrhythmia and cuts down hypertension. Research has also indicated that this mushroom enhances oxygen uptake by the brain and heart while improving resistance to hypoxia.

It is obvious from the range of scientific data which supports the many effective uses of *Cordyceps sinensis*. The herb has an important place in Chinese medicine and an increasing demand in the Western world for the alleviating of many conditions as well as for the strengthening of the body's functions in many ways. Such a diverse set of biological functions only adds credence to the multi-functional properties of this tonic herb.

How to Select the Best Source of Cordyceps Sinensis

What sort of herb is *Cordyceps sinensis*? It is, in fact, a parasitic fungus belonging to the major class of fungi called Ascomycetes. The fungus is found growing on the caterpillar larvae of Hepialus armoricanus belonging to the order of Lepidoptra—the butterflies and moths. If you purchased some *Cordyceps sinensis* from a Chinese apothecary, prior to 1985, you would probably have been given a bag of dried caterpillars and told to take 9 grams a day. Amazingly, people did get results from this unpurified source.

Due to its limited availability, Cordyceps is rather expensive, considerably higher than forms of ginseng. Although in recent years, its availability has improved in markets in Southeast Asia, Japan, and the U.S., demand still outweighs supply. Scientific studies have been done on *Cordyceps sinensis* since the 70s. Technological advances have allowed for the cultivation of Cordyceps in the laboratory. The fungus contains not only an abundance of nutrients (amino acids, vitamins, trace elements) but also active agents such as polysaccharides. Since 1985, the Chinese government has successfully cultivated the mycelia of Cordyceps sinensis in tissue culture and it is now not uncommon to find commercial preparations with hundreds of milligrams of pure mycelial extracts (Yin and Tang, 1995). This is by far the best source of Cordyceps sinensis and most likely to have the largest therapeutic effect. In fact, laboratory cultivation of has been so successful that it will likely completely replace natural Cordyceps in supplement form.

If your Cordyceps product is a listed therapeutic with the TGA, this is even better. At least under these circumstances you are assured of the manufacturing process and that the Cordyceps source meets an acceptable quality and purity. There have been recent reports of Cordyceps available from Chinese apothecaries that were heavily contaminated with toxic trace metals like lead and cadmium. In several cases this has led to lead poisoning (Wu, 1996). Check the label for any information you may need.

Complementary Herbs

Ginseng

Panax ginseng, or red ginseng, is another herb used for centuries in traditional medicine in China, reported to enhance stamina and the increase the ability to cope with stress and fatigue. There is an extensive body of research that deals with the biological functions of ginseng. The major active ingredients are the many saponins—steroid like substances—and the ginsenosides.

The ninety-five different ginsenoside saponins have also been shown to affect the neuroendocrine system , glucose and lipid metabolism, immune function and cardiac output. Many of the reports are based on animal studies with few human studies relating to performance enhancement or endurance availability. Yamasaki (1996), studied the effect of ginsenosides on the cellular uptake and utilization of glucose and found that they were strong activators of glucose transport and hence have a hypoglycemic effect.

Another recent study has shown that the organ protective actions of ginseng are linked to an enhanced production of nitric oxide (NO) by the vascular system, lungs, heart, kidney and brain. Nitric oxide is an important free radical produced in the body by a large number of different cells. The functions of NO are surprisingly extensive; it regulates platelet function, is a neurotransmitter, is involved in the regulation of immunity, inflammation and has an important role in vasodilatation and the elimination of intracellular pathogens. It is also responsible for the angina reducing effects of nitroglycerine. This effect on NO production could contribute to the vasodilatation and the aphrodisiac properties that have been reported for ginseng (Gillis,1997).

Studies by Fulder (1981), clearly demonstrated that ginseng saponins increase the sensitivity of the hypothalamic-pituitary-adrenal axis. This was demonstrated by an increase in corticosteroid binding in rat brains, which altered behavior and the response to stress. Bahrke and Morgan evaluated the ergogenic (or energy producing, fatigue reducing) properties of ginseng in 1994 and their review highlighted the lack of human studies in the area of performance. They did however point out that animal studies have shown clearly that the active components of ginseng do prolong the survival of animals exposed to extended physical and chemical stress.

One of the few human studies in ergogenic enhancement, using oral ginseng, did not find any ergogenic effects. The study measured a number of physical parameters during and after a cycle ergometer controlled ride. No significant difference between the placebo group and the ginseng group was observed with blood glucose, lactate, VO2 and RQ (respiratory quotient) (Morris et al, 1996).

The participants, however, were only give either 8 (approx. 550 mgs/day) or 16mg/kg (approx. 1100 mgs/day) for 7 days prior to the trial and this may have affected results as the normal TCM dosage is between 5 and 25 grams. Although a further study with oral administration of either 200 or 400 mgs/day for 8 weeks using graded maximal aerobic exercise as the measure, also showed on ergogenic effect with Panax ginseng (Engels and Wirth, 1997).

The other important nonsaponin constituent of ginseng is its antioxidant substance, Maltol. This powerful antioxidant is the principle that has been shown to improve central nervous system (CNS) activity and is the major contributor to the anti-aging, anti-irradiation, liver protection and anti-atherosclerosis effects associated with the use of ginseng (Huang, 1993). Maltol has a structure very closely related to vitamin E and hence is a very effective protective agent for cardiac and brain tissue. A clinical trial in involving healthy males, given oral ginseng for 9 weeks, showed a substantial lowering of heart rate when compared to the controls.

Panax ginseng would appear to have a number of properties that could benefit endurance and stamina but a major problem exists in that it is not easy to obtain standardized, authentic ginseng root preparations.

Ciwujia

Probably the most publicized and trendy endurance and stamina enhancing herbal supplement in the marketplace today is Endurox™. It is a standardized extract of ciwujia also known as *Acanthopanax senticosis, Eleutherococcus senticosis*, or Siberian ginseng. This herb is used as a ginseng substitute because of its low cost and wide availability. In Japan it is known as either Shigoja or Ezoukogi depending on locality and the part of the herb used.

The ciwujia saponin glycosides have powerful ginseng like effects. Ciwujia has been reported to stimulate the ACTH-cortisol system, lower blood pressure and blood glucose levels, enhance male sexual function, have a tranquilizing effect on the CNS and relieve stress (Huang, 1993). The Acanthosides of ciwujia have been shown to be powerful immunostimulating substances a property that is extremely important for OS and CF.

Animal studies with ciwujia have demonstrated that its extracts are extremely powerful in protecting against reperfusion induced arrhythmias, fibrillation and tachycardia (Tian et al., 1989). It has also been shown to be a powerful inhibitor of histamine release, an important feature in relation to performance injury (Umeyama et al., 1992). A number of studies have shown that ciwujia is extremely effective in protecting against exhaustion in a rat swimming stress model (Nishibe et al., 1990; Fujikawa et al., 1996). This is where the interest in this Chinese herb really has its beginnings.

A human study conducted by the University of North Texas Health Science center using a low intensity treadmill exercise protocol found that, with a supplementation of 1200 mg/day and after a 10 minute exercise at 8.5 kph, there was a considerable reduction in RQ which translated to a 22% increase in fat metabolism. Another study demonstrated that after administration for several weeks the accompanied drop in heart rate during prolonged exercise (up to 60 minutes) from 147 (control) to 137 (ciwujia treated) resulted in a 30% increase in fat metabolism with the oxygen intake per heartbeat during exercise being increased by 4.62% and 13% during recovery over the control group.

One of the more popular uses of ciwujia is in the treatment of chronic fatigue syndrome (CFS). Although a newly defined illness, CFS has been around a long time. Chronic fatigue syndrome can be a debilitating illness characterized by persistent fatigue along with other symptoms including low-grade fever, frequent sore throats, joint and muscle pain, and various neuro/psychological symptoms such as depression. Central to CFS is a disturbed immune system. While research has focused on trying to identify a specific infectious organism, CFS is more likely due to a general immune system failure.

Effective treatment of CFS must be comprehensive and address underlying factors that contribute to the weakened status of the immune system. However, ciwujia appears to address the fatigue, decreased sense of well-being, and impaired immune functions.

Ciwujia has been shown to exert a number of beneficial effects that may be useful in the treatment of CFS. In one double-blind study, thirty-six healthy subjects received either 10 ml of a ciwujia extract or placebo daily for 4 weeks. The group receiving the ciwujia fluid extract demonstrated significant improvement in a variety of immune system parameters. Most notable were a significant increase in helper T-cells and an increase in natural killer cell activity. Both of these effects could be put to good use in the treatment of chronic fatigue system.

Conclusion

Looking for the herbs and/or supplementation that will give you what you want—more energy or endurance through immune strengthening—can still be difficult. There continues to be some confusion in the literature and problems associated with the supply of some of the herbal endurance enhancers. However, there are some well-established approaches that can help you get that little bit closer to achieving an optimal level of health and energy.

For endurance and performance, branched chain amino acids, glutamine, magnesium, creatine monohydrate and choline are all well accepted. The amino acids help with anabolism and can protect against OS. Magnesium is a muscle protectant and a number of studies have shown it to help with recovery. Creatine loading has been well documented as an ergogenic enhancer. It has been shown to increase anaerobic capacity and the energy buffering capacity of the muscle (Brannon et al., 1997; Jacobs et al., 1997). Choline is a precursor for neurotransmitters, and it has been established that endurance workouts deplete choline stores leading to a significant fall in plasma choline levels by

50%. Taking choline can improve the performance of athlete's by 5 minutes over a 30 km run.

As this booklet shows, research supports that supplementing with *Cordyceps sinensis* can strengthen your immune system, which will help your body perform better in many ways. You'll have more energy and endurance as well as be able to fight off certain kinds of disease. Additionally, many negative conditions inside your body will be improved due to the influences of *Cordyceps sinensis* on the free radical cycle. All of these benefits are encompassed in the Chinese traditional explanation of what *Cordyceps sinensis* does for the body: It balances the forces within the body and strengthens the source of vitality. However you describe the action of this helpful herb, taking it can only benefit you and your health.

References

Bahrke and Morgan in 1994. Sports Med, Vol 18(4): pp 229-248.

Brannon et al, 1997. Med. Sci Sports Exerc. Vol. 29 (4). : pp489-495.

Chen J-R et al, 1993. American J. Chin. Med. Vol. XXI, Nos. 3-4: pp 257-262.

Cheng Q , 1992. Chung Hua Hseuh I Tsa-Chih (Tapei) Vol 72 (1) : pp27-29.

Engels HJ and Wirth JC, 1997. J Am. Diet Assoc. Vol 97 (10): pp1110-1115.

Fujikawa et al, 1996. Biol. Pharm. Bull Vol 19 (9) : pp1227 - 1230.

Fulder SJ, 1981. Am J Chin Med Vol. 9(2) : pp 112-118.

Gillis, CN, 1997. Biochem. Pharmacol. Vol. 54 (1): pp1-8.

Huang K C, 1993. The Pharmacology of Chinese Herbs. CRC Press Inc, USA..

Jacobs et al, 1997. Canadian Journal of Applied Physiol. Vol 22(3) : pp321-243.

Kletzien T F, 1980. Biochemical J. Vol 192 (2) : pp 753-759.

Kuo, WJ Tsai, M-S Shia, C-F Chen and C-Y Lin. American Journal of Chinese Medicine, Vol XXIV, No 2, pp 111-125.

Kuo Yuh-Chi et al, 1994. Cancer Investigation, Vol 12 (6): pp 611-615.

Kuo Yuh-Chi et al, 1996. Am J Chin Med., 24(2): 111-25, 1996.

Manabe, N. et al, 1996. Jpn J Pharamcol, 70(1):85-8, 1996 Jan

Mazumder A et al, 1995. Biochem. Pharmacol. Vol 49(8): pp1165-1170.

Montefiori DC et al, 1989. Proc. Natl. Acad. Sci. Vol. 86: pp 7191 - 7194.

Muller WEG et al, 1991. Biochemistry. Vol 30 : pp2027 - 2033.

Nishibe et al, 1990. Chem Pharm Bull Vol 38 (6) : pp 1763-1765.

Syrov VN, Nasyrova SS, and Khushbaktova ZA, 1997. Eksp Klin Farmakol Vol. 60 (3) : pp 41 - 44.

Tang R J et al, 1986. Chin. Trad. Herbal Drugs. Vol 17 : pp 22-25.

Tian et al, 1989. Chung Kuo Chung Yao Tsa Chih, Vol 14(8): pp493-495.

Taguchi T. et al, 1985. Japan. J Cancer Chemotherapy. Vol 12 : pp 366 - 375.

Ukai, S et al, 1996. Biol Pharm Bull, Vol. 19(2): pp 294-6.

Umeyama et al., 1992. J Pharma. Sci Vol 81(7) : pp 661-662.

Wu T N, 1996. Sci. Total Environ. Vol 182, (1-3) : pp193-195.

Xu H, Cheng,X and Wang, B. 1991. Chung Kuo Chung Yao Tsa Chih Vol. 16 (4) : pp237-240.

Yamasaki K, 1996. In Saponins used in Traditional and Modern Medicine, eds. Waller G.R. and Yamasaki, K. Vol 404, Advances in Experimental Medicine and Biology.Plenum Press, NY.

Yin D and Tang X, 1995. Chung Kuo Chung Yao Tsa Chih, Vol 20 (12) : pp707 -709.

Zhen F, 1992. Chung-Kuo-Chung His-I Chieh-Ho Tsa-Chih Vol 12 (4) : pp 207 209.